Gluten is my catalyst for a mental breakdown into a PTSD moment

Gluten complicates the relationship with illness such as Post Traumatic Stress Disorder (PTSD), Insomnia, plus other critical conditions.

Table of Contents

Printed in the United States of America
ISBN: 978-0-692-42963-1

Dedication

I dedicate this book to my mother, Anne Marie. Through no fault of her own, was stricken with the most confusing and heartbreaking illness. It has been my sole effort and joy, using my own will and determination to find out what happened to her life.

It is through this effort that I have been able to provide my mother's grandchildren with an explanation. This book is written for Christina and Elizabeth, who should never have to suffer through misdiagnosis as a way to live their lives.

Finally, my hope is to reach those people who need this information in their own lives, (no matter what their age) to make better choices for themselves. The decisions they make early on can lead to a much more stable and enjoyable life.

Disclaimer

The information presented in this book concerning gluten and the effect it has on the body has been obtained from authentic and reliable sources. Although great care has been taken to ensure the accuracy of the information presented, the author cannot assume responsibility for the validity of all the materials or the consequences for their use. Before starting diet changes or any regimen of vitamins or supplements, you should consult with your physician.

Introduction

The Dreams that Led Me to University of Minnesota Biomed Library

They repeated over and over. I was walking between all red brick buildings, concrete walkway underneath. The image was comfortable and serene, always a sunny day. I would walk lost for a time but always ended up in an area of lots of hallways, corridors, walking inside then outside following paths, then back inside again. I finally reached a place where everything was blue, sapphire blue.

Then one day in 2009, I was instructed travel to downtown Minneapolis and go to the Central Library. As I worked with a librarian there, she informed that the materials I was looking for was at the Biomed Library at U of M. It is open to the public so I will find what I'm looking for there.

I was instructed to get on a bus, it isn't necessary to drive. So I did. I called ahead to the bus company to find out which buses I needed. As it turned out, there was a city bus straight from my area directly to U of M. Reached the campus with all the kids in college, realizing I had never set foot on this campus before. Luckily, I was dropped off at Coffman Hall on the west bank, the Union Hall for campus, where an information booth was occupied. The young woman got a map and circled where I needed to be. Upon walking out the back door of Coffman Hall, I noticed I was walking between all red brick buildings, concrete walkways on a clear and sunny day. I wound my way over to the East Bank of which I have no remembrance of the path I took. Eventually I ended up at Mayo Complex which includes the Biomed Library.

I remember this next part clearly. Upon walking into the library, which is a couple of floors down, the carpeting is all blue, a sapphire blue. The librarian was so courteous, getting me signed onto a computer with her login information and introducing me to PubMed, the website of the US National Institute of Health. It was at this library that I could research keywords and have access to all the medical publications which I could copy to a flash card. It was the most incredible moment of my life. I am not a researcher or a medical professional. Yet I was sitting at the U of M, in the midst all the medical students and saying to myself "how in the world did I end up here". The librarian even asked me which do I prefer "PC or Mac".

One of the conditions that caught my attention was how much information was readily available, if you knew where to look. The Medical illustrations provided by Dr. Netter were produced in 1953-1976 timeframe. An example of his illustrations and the potential allergens is included in the book. The point I'm examining from Dr. Netter's work is the indication the allergic reaction originates in the mind. The point I'm making is the allergic reaction originates elsewhere in the body (see **Section "*PTSD is Born.*"**) My book goes on further to state how and why the intestines are broken down over time by ingesting gluten, thus setting the stage for additional serious illnesses to develop. My research unexpectedly led me to the work of Dr. Russell Blaylock, a board-certified Neurosurgeon and his experiences with neurodegenerative diseases, and the blood-brain barrier that gave me the resolve to write this book.

Best of Health and Good Reading.
Genevieve

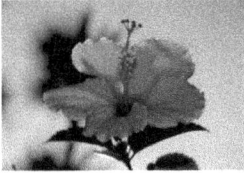

I shall attempt to summarize the 12 years of my mother's depression in the matter of the next few minutes. I would like to share with you the concerns of a family struggling with illness masquerading as depression but is actually Celiac's Disease or any variation of the condition that involves the intestines and immune system. I feel I can best relate this to you by telling my story, watching an unknown disease take hold in my life, yet with no understanding from doctors or even family members, as to what was happening. What I hope to accomplish is to present the medical information and research that I uncovered during my years trying to find answers as to what happened to her and for me.

It is my hope to share the information with those who are interested and want to prevent the same type of destruction and misdiagnosis happening in their lives. What I uncovered is far more sinister than I ever realized. I believe Celiac's Disease, Gluten Sensitivity or any allergies of the intestines in conjunction with parasitic invasion are the conditions that make the body ripe for catastrophic diseases in later years. I am referring to Parkinson's and Alzheimer's disease.

I can tell you that it is a sickness that never ends. My mother was a beautiful, smart woman, active in scouting with her children as well as a devout Catholic. A great tragedy, to be sure, for her children to watch their mother suffer from, what I consider to be an illness: Celiac's Disease. Watching the physical as well as mental deterioration take its toll on a vibrant, well-humored mother whose time with her children was cut short, is something I want to prevent in others. She was treated for Depression, Anxiety, Fear, Irrational Outbursts, and Emotional Disturbances. She was treated with every kind of anti-depressant made at the time, garbage bags full of prescription drugs, never even getting close to the source of the problems. As for myself, I have spent most of my adult years unraveling this personal medical mystery.

I am Gluten Sensitive. I feel compelled to tell my story because I believe it's my mother's story also. I believe she had a much weaker digestive system than other people, as I do. I believe years of financial stress that she endured and as I have, put an enormous strain on her which weakened her intestines and created the conditions for depression. But it was her excessive sleeping during the day and nightly insomnia that went on for years that brought this story home for me. I am her daughter and I shared her insomnia, if not variations of all her symptoms. It is because of the insomnia connection and constant tiredness that started this journey to find answers. I brought Celiac's disease/Gluten Sensitivity into the picture and am attempting to connect it all. It is with this reasoning that I proceeded to do my research.

I developed insomnia early in my life. I never connected my sleep problems with her sleep problems because no doctor ever said anything about them. She couldn't sleep well at night, then slept way too long during the day. In my case, I just couldn't sleep soundly and then was always tired the next day. I just accepted it. As my life progressed and I experienced much the same in the way of financial stress, my insomnia became worse. It was at this time that fear started to take over. I didn't know what was happening to me, why I couldn't sleep. I started to see similarities with my mother and it scared me.

The insomnia I experienced was an allergic reaction taking place in my intestines caused by Gluten. I had decided a long time ago, that if I started going down the path of my mother, I would explore all avenues of healing. Well, I had insomnia. I set out on another medical path into Traditional Chinese Medicine (TCM). One of the first recommendations listed for insomnia under TCM was to remove Gluten. However, insomnia is only one of many symptoms caused by Gluten, such as ADD/ADHD, even Autism in extreme cases. I was lead to Leaky Gut Syndrome (small holes or permeability in the intestines) after learning about Gluten as well as the overuse of antibiotics and its effects on the intestines.

Furthermore, I believe this is what my mother started out with early on in her illness, when her insomnia started. Celiac's Disease and/or Gluten Sensitivity is primarily a sensitivity to Gluten, proteins found in wheat, barley and rye. When people with Celiac Disease eat gluten, an allergic reaction takes place creating inflammation in the intestines which leads to permeability in the intestine walls. But she was never tested for Gluten allergies; she was treated for depression, the state of mind that is created by Gluten allergy. (There are other food allergens that need to be presented, more on this later.) She never went to a gastro-enterologist for depression. They, the psychiatrists, never found Gluten. Gluten proteins have even been linked to certain forms of schizophrenia. I believe she died at an early age because of all the years of misdiagnosis and incorrectly prescribed drugs. They took a toll on her body and mind. With her delicate constitution, she never stood a chance.

Leaky Gut Syndrome is the weakening of the intestines that leaks by small holes and allows toxins, parasites and undigested food particles into the bloodstream and take up residence within various organs, such as the appendix, liver, kidney and the brain, just to name a few.

Stress, in conjunction with Gluten, are the key ingredients that make the whole disease structure take place It is these very same holes that allow toxins and parasites to enter the body from food, water or particles in the air we breathe, to now have free reign over all bodily functions including the brain causing depression. I also believe Leaky Gut Syndrome is the portal by which other toxins, such as MSG and aspartate (also known as NutraSweet®), gain entry to the bloodstream and enter the brain through the Blood-Brain Barrier. It is through this sequence of events that, I believe, Alzheimer's and/or Parkinson's disease

11

begins its life within someone's brain, spine or has the potential to do so.

I am attempting to state facts so that you may better understand the effects of Celiac's Disease/Gluten sensitivity on my life and if you are reading this, perhaps your life. What I plan to accomplish with this writing is present the actions of the American Medical Community in the complete failure to diagnosis my mother's condition accurately resulting in her pain and suffering during her long-term illness which resulted in her death. Additionally, I hope to present how Celiac's Disease/Gluten Sensitivity can further affect a person's health, well into old-age. In the end, it was Her Creator that ultimately took her at an early age. Because if Alzheimer's or Parkinson's were the next stops on this already horrific train ride, then He undoubtedly spared all of my family, including my mother, from further pain and anguish at the hands of the American Medical Community.

Compiling this information has given me the strength, clarity and focus as to what happened during my life and to my Mother's life. It is through this awareness that I have found peace. Thank You

How Traditional Chinese Medicine (TCM) Helped:

A significant process I had to understand at the very beginning was the flow and timeline of food as it enters my body and exits my body. I ate beets because they exit the body beet red. It's a very useful method. I would write down what time and date I ate beets and what time and date they vacated my body. I'm on a 36 hour digestion clock. In other words, it takes 36 hours approximately for food to reach my lower intestines. This is where most of my allergies to food take place. My digestion path starts in the stomach, moves into upper GI tract (approximately 12 hours.) The food then moves into lower GI tract, (approximately 24 hours.) Finally, digested food moves into rectum and exit (approximately 36 hours). I don't know if my digestion body clock is fast, slow or normal. It is normal for my situation.

By knowing my digestion body clock, I could sync up with TCM Insomnia guidelines below as to what I ate 36 hours before I wake up in the middle of the night approximately 36 hours later (or anywhere in-between).

I was able to handle some of my own health care while continuing to work with my medical doctors. In this way, I was able to enhance my overall health strengthening healthy organs which propped up my kidneys ensuring continuing stable health for as long as possible. I don't know what the future brings for me and my kidneys, but I am doing everything possible for myself based upon a variety of medical sources, not just pharmaceutical (which is a necessary piece of the good health puzzle, but not the entire puzzle.)

American Medicine has revealed the same awareness to healing as Chinese Medicine. This is wonderfully documented by Jeffry Anderson, MD, Optimal Digestive Health, Chapter 13, "How Problems with Digestion Can cause Illness anywhere in the Body", Page 115.

> *"The presence of conditions caused by leaky gut syndrome indicates that toxins have been released from the GI tract and are out in general circulation. Then degenerative diseases such as cancer or autoimmune conditions can eventually develop."* -----Jeffry Anderson, M.D., Optimal Digestive Health, Page 116.

(Please Note: reading information presented by Traditional Chinese Medicine takes a little getting used to; there will be word combinations unfamiliar to most Americans. But pushing on through the written material is how you can find new and improved solutions.)

Insomnia and Traditional Chinese Medicine (TCM)

It was through the book "Healing with the Herbs of Life" by Lesley Tierra that I could take hold of overall health and my insomnia. Ms. Tierra put forth the following outline:

> *"Awake 11pm-3am: ...unable to fall asleep during this time or wake up now and can't fall back asleep.... Be sure to eliminate Liver-congesting foods such as caffeine, alcohol, dairy, {gluten}, nuts and nut butters...among others."*

> *"Awake 1am-3am or 3am-5am time slots: ...sleeplessness from indigestion can occur at this time...[and] is burdened by stagnation in the Large Intestines, ...resulting in...restless sleep and insomnia. Improve digestion, check for leaky gut syndrome...and take digestive [enzymes] during the day.*

14

If you are suffering from Insomnia during the 1am-3am or the 3am-5am time slot, be sure to eliminate food listed under "Foods to Avoid" as detailed in the same book. Possible food allergens such as dairy, eggs, gluten grains (wheat, oats, rye) corn, beans (especially soy), sugar and nuts is a basic outline of what TCM has to offer as helpful, useful information that works. This book is also a good introduction to Chinese Herbal medicine.

(See Section on Insomnia for more information)

Parkinson's and Alzheimer's Disease

It is my hope to share the information with those who are interested and want to prevent the same type of destruction and misdiagnosis happening in their lives. What I uncovered is far more sinister than I ever realized. I believe Celiac's Disease, Gluten Sensitivity or any allergies of the intestines in conjunction with parasitic invasion are the conditions that make the body ripe for catastrophic diseases in later years. I am talking about Parkinson's and Alzheimer's disease. (More on this topic will be presented in a later section.)

"The crucial point, however, is that gluten-sensitivity can also be associated with neurological symptoms in patients who do not have any mucosal gut damage (that is, without celiac disease). Gluten can cause neurological harm through a combination of cross-reacting antibodies, immune complex disease". -----PubMed Results 1. Med Hypotheses. 2009 Sep;73(3):438-40. Epub 2009 Apr 29. The gluten syndrome: a neurological disease. Ford RP. The Children's Gastroenterology and Allergy Clinic, PMID 1946584

"The toxoplasmic organisms infiltrate along the blood vessels of the brain, producing a lymphocytic and granulomatous response with subsequent areas of neucrosis cystic cavities and ventricular dilation...." ----- Netter, Frank H. MD., "The Ciba Collection of Medical Illustrations", CIBA, 1953

"These results suggest that Toxoplasma infection may be involved in the pathogenetic mechanisms of PD. If confirmed, this hypothesis would represent a valuable advancement in care of patients with Parkinson's disease". -----Pubmed Neurosci Lett, 2010 May 21; 475(3); 129-31 Epub 2010 Mar 27 The probable relation

between Toxoplasma Gondii and Parkinson's disease. PMID 20350582

"The real damage done...is to the intestinal epithelial barrier, allowing the absorption of serious toxic agents and chemicals, which then enter the blood and affect numerous organs, including the brain".-----Jake Paul Fratkin, OMD, Leaky Gut Syndrome, [Intestinal Barrier and the Blood-Brain Barrier] About Jake Paul Fratkin: He is nationally board-certified in both acupuncture and Chinese herbal medicine.

One of my greatest fears is that my own PTSD suffering, which comes and goes, is setting up a fragility within me that is happening now. I recently uncovered some research that suggests:

"...studies have found that those who suffer from posttraumatic stress disorder (PTSD) are more likely to experience dementia as they age, most often Alzheimer's disease (AD). These findings suggest that the symptoms of PTSD might have an exacerbating effect on AD progression". -----J Neurosci. 2015 Feb 11;35(6):2612-23. doi: 10.1523/JNEUROSCI.3333-14.2015. PMCID: PMC4323535 [Available on 2015-08-11]; PMID: 25673853 [PubMed – in process]

If this is true and NCBI's and the authors of the study are correct, wouldn't it be helpful if American Medicine would start looking at the effects of gluten on the intestinal lining and the corresponding toxic attacks on the whole body, especially the brain?

Author information: [1]Institute of Molecular Medicine, Program in Neuroscience, and Huffington Center on Aging and Department of Human and Molecular Genetics, Baylor College of Medicine, Houston, Texas 77030, and Nicholas.J.Justice@uth.tmc.edu.

[2]Department of Human and Molecular Genetics, Baylor College of Medicine, Houston, Texas 77030, and Jan and Dan Duncan Neurological Research Institute at Texas Children's Hospital, Houston, Texas 77030.

[3]Department of Integrative Biology and Pharmacology, University of Texas Health Sciences Center, Houston, Texas 77030.

[4]Huffington Center on Aging and.

[5]Institute of Molecular Medicine.[6]Institute of Molecular Medicine, Program in Neuroscience, and.[7]Huffington Center on Aging and Department of Human and Molecular Genetics, Baylor College of Medicine, Houston, Texas 77030

Gluten is my catalyst for a mental breakdown into a PTSD moment

It's not just for the military! I always thought PTSD was for war veterans but apparently not in my case, it's for me too. The feelings I experienced in the afternoon after eating a tiny little piece of Communion bread goes something like this:

> *Since I had the day off, I went to Mass and took Communion. This Communion was a little square of actual bread, not the flat-pressed type (the flat-pressed type are equally bad), which turned into a horrible experience later same day. My morning went well but the afternoon took a decidedly horrible turn, because that's the amount of time it took the little piece of bread to move out of my stomach and into my intestines. I started noticing similarities in my gluten-reaction to Post Traumatic Stress Disorder. I never connected the two, because most books on the subject never connect a food allergy such as gluten as a trigger mechanism to set off a PTSD episode. That was something only for war veterans.*

Where have you ever read or heard gluten is a trigger for a PTSD moment. NO WHERE. I believe my sensitivity to gluten has been the trigger mechanism over all these years that kept me locked in a PTSD pattern of suffering, albeit, a subtle, low-grade version. I believe anybody experiencing a trauma at any point in their lives can slip into a "PTSD" moment at any time in their life, and in my case, triggered by eating or drinking anything with gluten. Beer is made from wheat and barley. Both contain gluten. Why can't they drink gluten-free beer instead?

PTSD and Alzheimer's

One of my greatest fears is that my own PTSD suffering, which comes and goes, is setting up a fragility within me that is happening now. I recently uncovered some research that suggests

> *"...studies have found that those who suffer from posttraumatic stress disorder (PTSD) are more likely to experience dementia as they age, most often Alzheimer's disease (AD). These findings suggest that the symptoms of PTSD might have an exacerbating effect on AD progression."* -----J Neurosci. 2015 Feb 11;35(6):2612-23. doi: 10.1523/JNEUROSCI.3333-14.2015. PMCID: PMC4323535 [Available on 2015-08-11]; PMID: 25673853 [PubMed – in process]

If this is true and NCBI and the authors of the study are correct, wouldn't it be helpful if American Medicine would start looking at the effects of gluten on the intestinal lining and the corresponding toxic attacks on the whole body, especially the brain?

Author information: [1]Institute of Molecular Medicine, Program in Neuroscience, and Huffington Center on Aging and Department of Human and Molecular Genetics, Baylor College of Medicine, Houston, Texas 77030, and Nicholas.J.Justice@uth.tmc.edu.

[2]Department of Human and Molecular Genetics, Baylor College of Medicine, Houston, Texas 77030, and Jan and Dan Duncan Neurological Research Institute at Texas Children's Hospital, Houston, Texas 77030.

[3]Department of Integrative Biology and Pharmacology, University of Texas Health Sciences Center, Houston, Texas 77030.

[4]Huffington Center on Aging and.[5]Institute of Molecular Medicine.[6]Institute of Molecular Medicine, Program in Neuroscience, and.[7]Huffington Center on Aging and Department of Human and Molecular Genetics, Baylor College of Medicine, Houston, Texas 77030

Can you imagine what it's like for the folks returning from tours of duty overseas and their intestinal lining is deteriorated from the stress of war exploding all around them. They are being set up for misdiagnosed mental disturbances and or suicidal thoughts to which there seems to be no cure.

Veterans of War and Violence

"Alcoholic survivors may be males with PTSD from combat or from violent incidents that resemble combat. We shouldn't stereotype by gender, but I must point out that the "caregiver burden" for the wife of the traumatized vet is usually different than the role of the husband of the victimized wife. The male veteran with PTSD has a greater likelihood of being angry, aggressive, uncommunicative, secretly embarrassed and difficult to reach than the female with PTSD. Partners of male veterans have been systematically studied. A collection of these studies by Drs. Calhoun and Wampler in the National Center for PTSD Clinical Quarterly includes the statement, "almost half of these women (partners) reported having felt on the verge of a nervous breakdown." Calhoun and Wampler caution, "Many veterans suffering from chronic PTSD are openly distrustful and may view the involvement of their partner (in therapy) as a threat." ---- Gift From Within, PTSD resources for Survivors and Caregivers: Partners with PTSD, Frank Ochberg, M.D.
http://www.giftfromwithin.org/html/partners.html

All military should be put on a gluten free diet while they are overseas in war situations and as part of the reintroduction back to civilian life program. Like I mentioned above, war vets usually drink beer...and it contains gluten. I believe they are triggering a PTSD moments by allowing the allergen gluten into their body by drinking beer, eating pizza, or anything including wheat.

A real concern of mine is the complexity for diagnosis Doctors face when dealing with citizens and military alike. There is research available that details just how complex proper diagnosis can be.

> *"The detection of malingered PTSD is made particularly challenging by the subjective nature of PTSD criteria and requires a thorough, systematic approach. The psychiatrist must gather and analyze evidence from the evaluation, clinical records, psychologic testing, third parties and other sources. Although some individuals may malinger PTSD to avoid criminal sanctions, the most common motivation for malingering PTSD is financial gain".* ----- Psychiatr Clin North Am. 2006 Sep;29(3):629-47. PubMed PMID: 16904503

I'm reading all the steps the psychiatrist must go through in order to reach a solid diagnosis. I want to think that medical personnel are solving PTSD complaints and not claiming the symptoms, in some cases, are all made up in veteran's heads.

Luckily, Dr. Jeffry Anderson, MD has something different to say about Doctors and their diagnosis: *"Doctors observe that some of these conditions resolve naturally as a result of clearing the GI tract and liver. When you clean up the upstream issues and the liver, then the downstream consequences tend to just go away."* ----Optimal Digestive Health, Page 117. Biographical information for Jeffry Anderson, MD appears on Page 86 Optimal Digestive Health.

"Distinguishing schizophrenia from post-traumatic stress disorder with psychosis [in returning Veterans]."

"Up to 70% of returning veterans experience symptoms of PTSD. These individuals also fall within the peak age range for the onset of schizophrenia. PTSD with psychosis may occur for several reasons: trauma increases one's risk for schizophrenia and PTSD; patients with schizophrenia have a higher incidence of PTSD and may present with characteristic psychotic symptoms overlapping with psychosis in schizophrenia".----PubMed ID:25785709

Please see section on **Gluten Proteins and Schizophrenia**.

I keep reading that PTSD is linked to many illnesses that affect returning Veterans, probably for the rest of their lives. If misdiagnosis is allowed to continue, then millions of lives will have experienced suffering way beyond the inflictions of wartime itself.

"RESULTS: A drastic reduction, if not full remission, of schizophrenic symptoms after initiation of gluten withdrawal has been noted in a variety of studies". -----
The gluten connection: the association between schizophrenia and celiac disease. Kalaydjian AE, Eaton W, Cascella N, Fasano A. Acta Psychiatr Scand 2006 Feb; 113(2): 82-90 PMID 16423158 PubMed

"Sleep Problems may mediate associations between rumination and PTSD and depressive symptoms among OIF/OEF veterans."

"Operation Iraqi Freedom/Operation Enduring Freedom (OIF/OEF) veterans have high rates of posttraumatic stress disorder (PTSD), depression, and sleep problems....Rumination or repeated thoughts about negative experiences, is associated with worse PTSD, depression, and sleep problems....Additionally, we [PubMed Authors] propose a novel hypothesis that sleep problems are a mechanism by which rumination contributes to depressive and PTSD symptoms".----PMID 25793596, Psychol Trauma 2015, Jan 7(1): 76-84

Keep in mind, the above-referenced hypothesis does not mention what is causing the sleep problems. What this quote appears to be stating is that the sleep problems begin in the mind through ruminating thoughts. What **MY** hypothesis is stating is that gluten is an allergen that directly impacts sleep by way of incomplete digestion once gluten enters the GI tract. At that moment, sleep is disturbed and the individual awakens as he or she progresses through the various sleep stages outlined in Traditional Chinese Medicine (TCM). Please see the section on ***Insomnia and Traditional Chinese Medicine.*** It is clear to me from my own experience that sleep problems are a result of an allergic reaction caused by gluten taking place within the digestive tract. It is from that food irritation that causes my own ruminations, hence the title of this book: "Gluten is My catalyst for a mental breakdown into a PTSD moment." All of which contribute to depressive and PTSD symptoms. This is most apparent during 1:00am sleep cycle. It's the middle of the night and I'm wide awake. I *always* know its gluten, because it's always the same time, give or take ½ hour or so. Even if I'm extremely careful with what I eat, there is so much hidden gluten in food manufacturing today it's exhausting. For example, food preparer's don't always know what's in some items labeled "Natural Flavors". I am forced to call each and every manufacturer of products I buy to make sure there is no "hidden gluten".

Dr. Netter and his diagram had everything right except that the effects of gluten originate in the intestines and circle back around affecting the brain. PTSD is born. Clean up the GI Tract and this issue may resolve itself.

Please Note: The allergens as detailed have been known since 1953 through 1976. -----F. Netter, MD, "Intestinal Disturbances Due to Psychic Factors, Allergy and Endogenous Infection", The Ciba Collection of Medical Illustrations, Digestive System, CIBA-GEIGY Corporation, 1953-1976

Insomnia Connection

I believe years of financial stress that my Mother endured and as I have, put an enormous strain on her which weakened her intestines and created the conditions for depression. But it was her excessive sleeping during the day and nightly insomnia that went on for years that brought this story home for me. I am her daughter and I shared her insomnia, as well as variations of all her symptoms. It is because of the insomnia connection and constant tiredness that started this journey to find answers. I brought Celiac's disease/Gluten Sensitivity into the picture and am attempting to connect it all. It is with this objective that I proceeded to do my research.

> *"It is not uncommon to find disturbed ... patterns as the predominant presentation, marked by insomnia or restless sleep, anxiety, easily frightened, or palpitations. These are anxiety or anti-depressive medications. Chinese herbal medicine is quite effective here."* -----Jake Paul Fratkin, OMD, Leaky gut Syndrome, Part II: Heart and Shen Patterns

> *"...significant [financial] stress is almost always associated with mucosal erosions, particularly in the stomach. A majority of these lesions are subclinical, but gastrointestinal hemorrhage and sepsis are not infrequent consequences".* ----- http://arbl.cvmbs.colostate.edu/hbooks/pathphys/digesti on/stomach/gibarrier.html

I developed insomnia early in my life. I never connected my sleep problems with her sleep problems because no doctor ever said anything about them. She couldn't sleep well at night, then slept way too long during the day. In my case, I just couldn't sleep soundly and then was always tired the next day. I just accepted it. As my life progressed and I experienced much the same in the way of financial stress, my insomnia became worse. It was at this time that fear started to take over. I didn't know what was happening to me, why I couldn't sleep. I started to see similarities with my mother and it scared me.

The insomnia I experienced was an allergic reaction taking place in my intestines caused by Gluten. I had decided a long time ago, that if I started going down the path of my mother, I would explore all avenues of healing. Well, I had insomnia. I set out on another medical path into Traditional Chinese Medicine (TCM and/or Chinese Herbal Medicine). One of the first recommendations listed for insomnia under TCM was to remove Gluten.

Small Holes in the Intestines

However, insomnia is only one of many symptoms caused by Gluten, such as ADD/ADHD, even Autism in extreme cases. I was led to Leaky Gut Syndrome (small holes or permeability in the intestines) after learning about Gluten as well as the overuse of antibiotics and its effects on the intestines.

"A number of mental conditions have been linked to increased permeability. The elevated toxins that leak into the system from hyperpermeability can produce symptoms that range from spaciness and brain fog to attention deficit disorder. We now know that many children with ADD/ADHD have increased gut permeability. In the most extreme form hyperpermeability can cause disorientation resembling autism or schizophrenia. In some cases these disorders are also linked to specific food sensitivities such as gluten sensitivity. And a number of stresses can be affecting the body at once: Toxic load on the system appears to affect neurotransmitter production, and specific allergies may directly affect the nervous system as well. Recent research links some allergic responses with brain chemistry and reactions in the receptor sites (see Chapter 8)". -----Len Saputo, M.D., "Leaky Gut Syndrome-Other Factors", Optimal Digestive Health, Page 63

"Leaky Gut Syndrome (LGS) is a major cause of disease and dysfunction in modern society, and in my practice accounts for at least 50% of chronic complaints, as confirmed by laboratory tests. In LGS, the epithelium on the villi of the small intestine becomes inflamed and irritated, which allows metabolic and microbial toxins of the small intestines to flood into the blood stream. This event compromises the liver, the lymphatic system, and

the immune response including the endocrine system". ----Jake Paul Fratkin, OMD, Leaky Gut Syndrome, Part I, The Problem

"The presence of chronic gastrointestinal (GI) symptoms in children with autism spectrum disorder (ASD) has been well established. ...the frequency of these chronic and often intense GI symptoms, reveal that they occur in as many as 70-80% of ASD Children....In the [Author's] experience with ASD children, the following diagnoses have been endoscopically confirmed and determined to be causing some or all of these symptoms: ... CELIAC DISEASE, non-specific colitis, Crohn's disease". -----Arthur Krigsman, MD, "My Child Has Stomach Aches, Constipation, and Diarrhea. What Might the Problem Be and What Should I Expect from a Visit With the Gastroenterologist? Can These Problems Be Treated?" The Autism File, Pg. 14-18

"What modern event allowed such a break-down? Primarily it has been antibiotics, secondarily non-steroidal anti-inflammatory drugs (NSAIDs). The first antibiotic, penicillin, did not enter mainstream health care until 1939.... NSAIDs are commonly taken for various pains, and include ibuprofen (Motrin®, Advil®). They are quite damaging to the small intestine mucosa lining". ----Jake Paul Fratkin, OMD, Leaky gut Syndrome, Antibiotics Destroy Beneficial Bacteria

Gluten Proteins and Schizophrenia

Furthermore, I believe this is what my mother started out with early on in her illness, when her insomnia started. Celiac's Disease and/or Gluten Sensitivity is primarily a sensitivity to Gluten, proteins found in wheat, barley and rye. When people with Celiac Disease/Gluten Sensitivity eat gluten, an allergic reaction takes place creating inflammation in the intestines which leads to permeability in the intestine walls. But she was never tested for Gluten allergies; she was treated for depression, the state of mind that is created by Gluten allergy originating in the intestines. (There are other food allergens that need to be presented; *See Section PTSD is Born*...) She never went to a gastro-enterologist for depression. They, the psychiatrists, never found Gluten. Gluten proteins have even been linked to certain forms of schizophrenia.

"RESULTS: A drastic reduction, if not full remission, of schizophrenic symptoms after initiation of gluten withdrawal has been noted in a variety of studies". ----- The gluten connection: the association between schizophrenia and celiac disease. Kalaydjian AE, Eaton W, Cascella N, Fasano A. Acta Psychiatr Scand 2006 Feb; 113(2): 82-90 PMID 16423158 PubMed

Polycystic Kidney Disease (PKD)

Leaky Gut Syndrome is the weakening of the intestines that leaks by small holes and allows toxins, parasites and undigested food particles into the bloodstream and take up residence within various organs, such as the appendix, liver, kidney and the brain, just to name a few. I finally found the proof I have been looking for.

> *"Polycystic Kidney Disease: An Unrecognized Emerging Infectious Disease? assay [def: analysis] showed bacterial endotoxin and fungal ...in cyst fluids from human kidneys with PKD".*-----Emerging Infectious Diseases, Vol. 3, No. 2, April-June 1997

> *"The intestinal mucosa is a major barrier that functions to prevent bacteria colonizing the gut from invading systemic organs and tissues. Under certain conditions, bacteria normally confined to the gastrointestinal (GI) tract can cross this mucosal barrier and appear in the mesenteric lymph nodes (MLN) and other organs, a process termed bacterial translocation. Factors that promote the translocation of bacteria from the GI tract include disruption of the ecology of the indigenous GI micro flora leading to bacterial overgrowth, impaired host immunity, and physical disruption of the gut mucosal barrier."* -----
> "Endotoxin Promotes the Translocation of Bacteria from the Gut", Edwin A. Deitch, MD; Rodney Berg, PhD; Robert Specian, PhD, Arch Surg—Vol 122, Feb 1987

Alzheimer's, [Parkinson's], Lou Gehrig's disease (ALS) via the Blood-Brain Barrier

Stress, in conjunction with Gluten, are the key ingredients that make the whole disease structure take place   It is these very same holes that allow toxins and parasites to enter the body from food, water or particles in the air we breathe, to now have free reign over all bodily functions including the brain causing depression. I also believe Leaky Gut Syndrome is the portal by which other toxins, such as [parasites], MSG and aspartate (also known as NutraSweet®), gain entry to the bloodstream and enter the brain through the Blood-Brain Barrier. It is through this sequence of events that, I believe, Alzheimer's and/or Parkinson's disease begins its life within someone's brain, spine or has the potential to do so.

> *"For example, glutamate can cause widespread destruction of certain brain cells in concentrations normally found in the diet. This is especially so when we consider the enormous amounts of glutamate added to our food in the form of the taste enhancer, monosodium glutamate or MSG. Without the blood brain barrier this glutamate would do serious damage to the brain and spinal cord. But, this protection has certain limitations..."*-----Russell Blaylock M.D., The Blood Brain Barrier: Protecting the Brain, "Excitotoxins", Page 18

> *"...high levels of dietary Excitotoxins, such as MSG and aspartate, could greatly aggravate the condition and cause it to progress more rapidly".*-----Russell Blaylock M.D., Defective Energy Production in Alzheimer's Neurons, "Excitotoxins", Page 167 "ExcitoToxins - The Taste that Kills: How monosodium glutamate, aspartame (NutraSweet®) and similar substances can cause harm to the brain and nervous system and their relationship to

neurodegenerative diseases such as Alzheimer's, [Parkinson's], Lou Gehrig's Disease (ALS) and others."

Dr. Blaylock then goes on to say...

"Toxins are known to travel through the blood brain barrier to create Alzheimer's and/or traveling through the spinal blood barrier to create Parkinson's disease." ----- This information is coming from, Russell L. Blaylock, M.D. He is a board-certified neurosurgeon who completed his medical training at the Louisiana State University School of Medicine in New Orleans, Louisiana.

"However, the barrier is not perfect. In fact, some parts of the brain never develop a barrier system at all. For example, the hypothalamus, the circumventricular organs, the pineal, and a small nucleus in the brain stem called the locus ceruleus, are without barrier protection. There is also evidence that the barrier is broken down or at least partially malfunctioning under certain conditions."

"Experimentally, it has been shown that with prolonged exposure to high blood levels of glutamate and aspartate these Excitotoxins do seep past the blood-brain barrier and enter the brain. Under normal conditions most people are exposed to multiple foods and drinks containing MSG, hydrolyzed vegetable protein, and aspartate due to the widespread use of these taste enhancers by the food industry. In addition, we consume these foods and drinks all day long (as snacks as well as meals) and with each dose of glutamate the blood level of these Excitotoxins rises for many hours afterwards. This constant barrage of the brain's gatekeeper by Excitotoxins means that a significant amount could enter the brain and spinal cord."

-Russell Blaylock M.D., Failure of the Gatekeeper: The Blood-Brain Barrier, "Excitotoxins", Page 167-168" Excitotoxins - The Taste that Kills: How monosodium glutamate (MSG), aspartame (NutraSweet®) and similar substances can cause harm to the brain and nervous system and their relationship to neurodegenerative diseases such as Alzheimer's, [Parkinson's], Lou Gehrig's Disease (ALS) and others. "

Alzheimer's disease and PTSD

One of my greatest fears is that my own PTSD suffering, which comes and goes, is setting up a fragility within me that is happening now. I recently uncovered some research that suggests

> "...studies have found that those who suffer from posttraumatic stress disorder (PTSD) are more likely to experience dementia as they age, most often Alzheimer's disease (AD). These findings suggest that the symptoms of PTSD might have an exacerbating effect on AD progression." -----J Neurosci. 2015 Feb 11;35(6):2612-23. doi: 10.1523/JNEUROSCI.3333-14.2015. PMCID: PMC4323535 [Available on 2015-08-11]; PMID: 25673853 [PubMed – in process]

If this is true and NCBI's and the authors of the study are correct, wouldn't it be helpful if American Medicine would start looking at the effects of gluten on the intestinal lining and the corresponding toxic attacks on the whole body, especially the brain?

Author information: [1]Institute of Molecular Medicine, Program in Neuroscience, and Huffington Center on Aging and Department of Human and Molecular Genetics, Baylor College of Medicine, Houston, Texas 77030, and Nicholas.J.Justice@uth.tmc.edu.

[2]Department of Human and Molecular Genetics, Baylor College of Medicine, Houston, Texas 77030, and Jan and Dan Duncan Neurological Research Institute at Texas Children's Hospital, Houston, Texas 77030.

[3]Department of Integrative Biology and Pharmacology, University of Texas Health Sciences Center, Houston, Texas 77030.

[4]Huffington Center on Aging and.[5]Institute of Molecular Medicine.[6]Institute of Molecular Medicine, Program in Neuroscience, and.[7]Huffington Center on Aging and Department of Human and Molecular Genetics, Baylor College of Medicine, Houston, Texas 77030,

In Conclusion

American Medical Community

I am attempting to state facts so that you may better understand the effects of Celiac's Disease/Gluten sensitivity on my life and if you are reading this, perhaps your life. What I plan to accomplish with this writing is present the actions of the American Medical Community in the complete failure to diagnosis my mother's condition accurately resulting in her pain and suffering during her long-term illness which resulted in her death. Additionally, I hope to present how Celiac's Disease/Gluten Sensitivity can further affect a person's health, well into old-age. In the end, it was Her Creator that ultimately took her at an early age. Because if Alzheimer's or Parkinson's were the next stops on this already horrific train ride, then He undoubtedly spared all of my family, including my mother, from further pain and anguish at the hands of the American Medical Community.

> *"In terms of education, medical students and house officers, under the constant tutelage of industry representatives, learn to rely on drugs and devices more than they probably should [my emphasis]. As the critics of medicine so often charge, young physicians learn that for every problem, there is a pill [my emphasis] (and a drug company representative to explain it). They also become accustomed to receiving gifts and favors from an industry that uses these courtesies to influence their continuing education. The academic medical centers, in allowing themselves to become research outposts for industry, contribute to the overemphasis on drugs and devices."*-----
> T. Colin Campbell, PhD and Thomas M. Campbell II, "Big Medicine: Whose Health Are They Protecting? Hooked on Drugs", Page 334, The China Study

"The ego of these people is enormous. And then someone comes along and says, "You know, I think we can cure this with Brussel sprouts and broccoli." The doctor's response is, "WHAT? I learned all this crap, I'm making a freakin' fortune, and you want to take it all away?"-----T. Colin Campbell, PhD and Thomas M. Campbell II, "Big Medicine: Whose Health Are They Protecting? A Daunting Task" Page 325, The China Study

"I have now treated a number of senior staff with coronary disease at the Clinic--senior staff physicians. I have also treated a number of senior staff trustees. One of the trustees knows about the frustrations that we've had trying to get this into the clinic, and he says, "I think, if the word gets out that Esselstyn has this treatment that arrests and reverses this disease at the Cleveland Clinic, and it's been used by senior staff and he's treated senior trustees, but he's not permitted to treat the common herd, we could be open for a lawsuit."-----T. Colin Campbell, PhD and Thomas M. Campbell II, "Big Medicine: Whose Health Are They Protecting? Esselstyn's Reward" Page 340, The China Study

(Note from this Author): (The above-referenced quote is referring to coronary disease and they are talking about reversing heart disease through changing the diet. I feel this same argument can be applied to all diseases, especially reasons to be gluten-free.

Final Words...

Hi, my name is Genevieve Campbell and I'd like to tell you my present day story. Compiling this information has given me the strength, clarity and focus as to what happened during my life and to my Mother's life. It is through this awareness that I have found peace.

I am writing this as a way to introduce myself and what's happening to me now. I am a Polycystic Kidney Disease (PKD) patient yet I show no signs of illness, other than the numbers on my charts. My other organs are in fantastic shape. This is because I am gluten-free and have been for 9 years. I watch my diet very carefully and I watch my sleep very carefully. At some point, my Kidney Doctor suggested I visit and understand what the kidney transplant program was all about, just so I was prepared. You see, PKD worsens progressively as time goes on.

I was completely horrified at the options presented to me by the Transplant Center. The transplant medicines are not perfected. The dialysis option is outdated. At no time did they even mention progress being made in stem cell research or other areas in medicine. Most definitely, nothing was mentioned using Holistic Medicine and the ideas contained. Traditional Chinese Medicine is one example.

I felt there had been nothing new to offer me different from what was offered my mother 30 years prior. Over 30 Years, this is all I get! This is how I felt. I will wait because a transplant, if one is ever available for me, is no less than 5 years. I believe, hope and pray much progress will be made in area of Kidney Disease by then.

Contact Information:

Please email me with your questions or comments. I can't answer every one personally, but be assured that your comments mean very much to me and I thank you for taking the time to send them. You can Google Search my name "Genevieve Campbell" and leave me a comment on G$^+$. Otherwise email me at: 57chevyb@gmail.com

A Friend in Good Health,
Genevieve Campbell

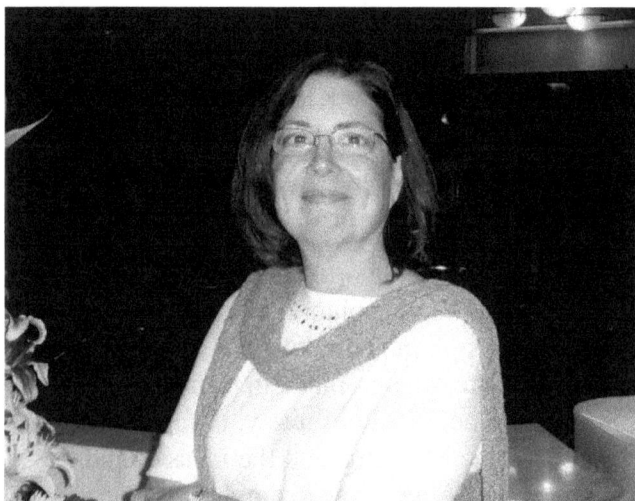

www.ingramcontent.com/pod-product-compliance
Lightning Source LLC
Chambersburg PA
CBHW060748280326
41934CB00010B/2404

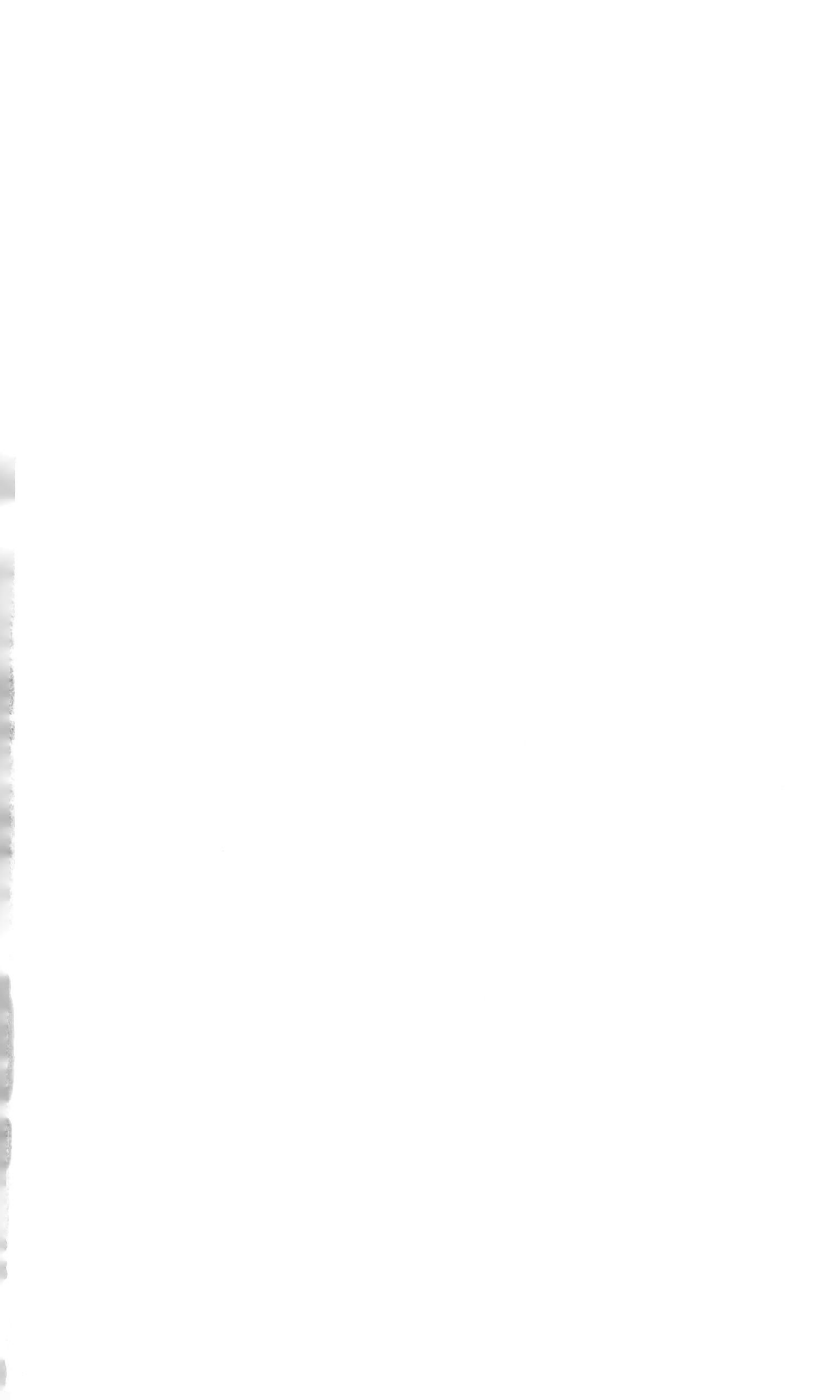